The Gift of
DIS·EASE

LORI TIDWELL

ISBN-13: 978-1542352895

ISBN-10: 1542352894

DISCLAIMER

This book is sold for information purposes only. Neither the author nor the publisher will be held accountable for the use or misuse of the contents of this book. This book is not intended as medical advice, and neither the author nor publisher of this work are medical doctors, and do not claim or make professional or medical recommendations on curing or treating any medical condition. Because there is always some risk involved with any activity, the author, publisher, and distributers will not be held liable for any adverse consequences concurrent or resultant from any suggestions or activities presented in this book. The reader is responsible to seek professional medical advice and make decisions regarding their own health.

TABLE OF CONTENTS

ACKNOWLEDGMENTS

I'd like to thank my family for their love and support, especially my husband Blaine and my four sons- Trevor, Jordon, Dallin, and Alec. They've been with me through good times and the crazy times. I love you!

I'd also like to thank dear friends and mentors who have been instrumental in my journey of healing- Becky Johnson, Sandra Boyer, Denise Silvernail, Dino & Shannon Watt, Annette Brandley, Lynda Smith, and Kirk Duncan. To my other life-long friends, you are simply the best!

Love & Gratitude,
Lori

INTRODUCTION

"If you focus on the problem, you can't see
the solution. Never focus on the problem... See
what no one else sees. See what everyone else
chooses not to see, out of fear, and conformity,
and laziness. See the whole world anew each day."
    -Arthur, "Patch Adams", 1998

Nine years ago, I woke up feeling like I
had the flu. I had a fever and a terrible
headache. I was sick and miserable. This
was becoming my new normal. I was tired
all of the time, and I wasn't being the kind
of wife, mother, or person I wanted. I felt
angry! I rolled over in my bed and looked
at the nightstand and all the medications on
it. There were eight of them. I thought,
"There has to be a better way to live. There

has got to be a better way to do this!" I sat up on my bed and began to cry uncontrollably.

In that moment I cried out to God, "I don't care if I have 5 more days or 50 more years to live, I don't want to spend one more day like this! What do I need to do?" An answer came immediately.

"Go off of all your medications. I'll show you what you can do." So I took a giant leap of faith. And that was the beginning of my journey, a journey which unfolded step by step, piece by piece, which led me to where I am today: living a healthier, happier, medication and symptom free life!

I hope you will be able to see your disease through different eyes; that you can learn to embrace your challenges by finding the gifts within them. There is more than one way to get what you want. I wanted to feel better. I wanted my life back – the life I had before illness, only BETTER! I have it. All of it, and more! I want it for you too. This book is about how I ended my struggle with chronic illness. Your journey may be different than mine. It may take you down different paths than mine, or it may be longer or shorter than mine, and that's alright. The similarities will be found in the guiding principles-the compass- that healed my life. They can be a compass for you too. I hope you find the gifts within your challenges, and that you experience joy in your journey!

I HAVE CHOICES

I have choices. I can choose in every moment what I do, what I say, what I think, how I feel, and how I act. Perception is a choice. How I perceive a person, place, or situation, is up to me.

I come from a very large and wonderful family and extended family. I am fortunate to have grown up knowing all of my grandparents and four of my great-grandparents. I am the oldest of 7 children; I have 1 brother and 5 sisters. My sisters and I love to sing together. We had our typical sibling issues growing up, but we are best friends now. I get together with my whole family a once a month. We eat dinner and just spend time with the whole crew. My parents have 24 grandchildren, so it is quite an undertaking. We enjoy connecting with each other and being together, however, there is one thing that we need to adjust when we get together, and that is the direction most of our conversations take. I've noticed a pattern: it seems like a lot of our conversations are about the struggles and problems we are having. We do take time to recognize the kids for their achievements, and the occasional update on someone feeling better after an injury or sickness, but the dominant topic of conversation is mostly about our problems. We sound like a real fun bunch to be around, don't we? That is sad to me, because we are a fun and passionate group of people to be around. I just asked the question, "What are we more passionate about, our struggles or our triumphs?"

When it came my turn to host the family get-together, I decided to shake things up a bit. I placed a "No Complaining Zone" poster on my front door with balloons. I gave smiley stickers to the girls to stick on people when they heard them engaging in positive conversations. After dinner, we gathered in the living room. Each person was given the opportunity to talk about something wonderful that had happened in their life within the previous week. A few people struggled to come up with something good to say, even as others came up with something quickly. It felt good to see my family talking positively about themselves and their lives. It is interesting how easy it can be for us to dwell on what's not going so well in our lives instead of the beauty and good that happens each day!

I see this when I interact with people who have chronic illness. It is fascinating to listen to a group of people try to outdo one another's 'woe-is-me' story, or see who has the greater hardship, or who is suffering the most, as if there is a prize for being the most put upon. I began to question my own belief about what my illness, multiple sclerosis, had to "look like" and my own tales of woe. How much power was I giving to them by repeating those stories over and over? I asked myself the question; Did I value my health and well-being more than I valued my victim story, or did I value my victim story more than my health? The answer was yes, I do value my health and well-being more than my 'woe-is-me' story. Do I have problems? Yes. Do those problems define me? No! I am not my challenges. I am not the disease I've been diagnosed with. The disease is an event happening in my life, not who I am. I have choices. I make decisions daily, hourly, minute by minute, about what kinds of experiences I will have.

I am grateful for the doctors who supported me when I chose to eliminate all of the medications I was on and seek "alternative" ways to heal myself. It was my path to take. The path you choose may be different. Am I cured? I suppose not, but what is "cured" anyway? MS was not the only thing I needed healing of. I needed to heal my mind and spirit. I needed to cure some false beliefs I had, which eliminated some of my symptoms in the process.

Disease can often be brought on from psychological stress. Stress comes from believing you don't have options, that something is being "done to you", or that you don't have any choice. By looking at MS though different lenses, I was able to see that it wasn't my body, so much, that needed healing. It was my heart and mind. I had all sorts of thoughts and beliefs that were damaging me, causing negative things in my body. Thoughts like: "I'm not good enough." "I'm stupid." "I never get things right." "Things never go my way." "I'm fat and ugly." "It works out for everyone but me." Yikes! I don't ever want to think or feel that way about myself again.

Have you ever felt like you keep repeating the same mistakes over and over? Have you ever thought, "What is wrong with me?" or "Why can't I get this right?" Is it a merry-go-round you'd like to stop? Have you ever uttered the words, "I should have known better?"

I was talking with a friend one day, telling her about a situation, when I said, "I should've known better."

She put her hand up and said "Stop! Who says? Is that a true statement?"

I paused for a few seconds searching my mind for an answer. She then continued to say, "I'm just betting you did the best thing you knew how to do in that situation, given the knowledge you had at that time."

She was right. I had done the best I knew how, in that situation. Are there things I may do differently if a similar situation comes up? Probably, because I have new information about what worked and what didn't work.

I have discovered that no good comes from trying to live life from a "would've, could've, should've" perspective. The truth is, I do the best I know how in any given situation. And the truth is, I can't change what has already happened. When I come from a "would've, could've, should've" perspective, it causes me to doubt and mistrust myself. I get stuck in a repeating cycle of self-doubt and mistrust- a cycle I want to stop repeating, because feeling stuck never feels good to me. So what do I do to get unstuck and free myself in order to move forward? First, I catch myself thinking those thoughts. Then I acknowledge that I did the best I knew how in that situation. Next, I ask myself what worked in that situation and what didn't work. I also ask myself what I would change to produce a better outcome. Then I do better next time with the new perspective and knowledge I have.

I find it interesting how some people react when they discover how I have put my MS so far back on the burner that I don't even really have it anymore. They often seem indifferent about it. They will act as if it's an interesting coincidence, or that I just "lucked out". The truth is, it is a big deal, and luck had nothing to do with it. I live free of symptoms, and free from medications, when I "should" be tired, in pain, or even bed-ridden. I am healthy because I have made the choice to find value in the challenges I face in my life. I don't identify with the disease at all. I have used the things I am sharing in this book to shift my perspective and my beliefs that are out of whack. I have changed my eating habits. I practice being grateful and forgiving every day. I reduce the stress in my life by doing all of these things. I became the hero in my life. Yet many people would rather chalk it up to luck, and get on commiserating about all of their problems and struggles, as if it is easier to struggle and endure the hardship. But not everyone reacts that way. People in real physical and emotional pain will catch a glimmer of hope and enthusiastically ask how I did it; people who are sick and tired of being sick and tired, who want to find their own "super powers" and create a healthy life. They "get it".

Not everyone is going to be on board with you making changes. Please realize that change, even good change, is challenging, not only for you but for those closest to you. When you make a choice to move out of your comfort zone, you'll often push the people you love out of their comfort zone as well. It's as though you decided to get on a rollercoaster ride and dragged everyone in your life along with you, whether they were ready or not! A few will buckle in, throw their hands up in the air and figure out how to enjoy the ride. Some will be scared, nervous, and a little ticked off, but will find some pleasure in the experience. The last few will be annoyed, angry and scared to their core.

Now while you're on this roller coaster ride, you get to decide how much, if any, of your power you are going to keep or give away, and to whom. Giving your power to someone else looks like you doubting yourself, you doubting your inner voice, doing what others tell you to just because they are in an "authority" position or "know more" than you. It's not acting on a gut feeling because of what others' may think about you, or conforming to the outside voices. It's giving in to stop people from feeling uncomfortable or trying to justify your decisions. It can also be constantly apologizing for your changes and new decisions. When you give any of your power to family members, friends, doctors, or anyone else, it will slow you down and make for a bumpier ride, and can even derail you at times. It doesn't mean all is lost; it just means you need to get back on track, using principles from this book and following your inner guide. You are not responsible for the type of experience everyone else is having on the roller coaster ride. It does make it so much better when you are compassionate and loving toward others, especially when you are the one that brought them on this ride in the first place!

I have experienced resistance from others as I have made changes, ones that improved my health, my spirituality, and my outlook on life for the better. Sometimes growth is painful, emotionally and physically, but it is so worth it.

I hope you awaken to the healing powers you possess within you. Don't let the simplicity fool you. By small and simple things, great things are brought to pass. Our bodies are wonders. Our bodies know how to heal.

As I was holding my niece an hour after she was born, I was pondering on that tiny little body that somehow knew how to do all it was supposed to- her heart knew how to beat, her mouth knew how to suck, her blood knew how to circulate, and her brain knew how to coordinate it all. It is truly amazing.

We must support our body with good nutrition and movement. We must support our mind with healthy thoughts, and eliminate belief patterns that hinder us instead of help us. Our spirit must be free to express its divinity and worth by letting go of burdens which render it unhealthy. I have choice, ability, and the power to change my story.

GRATITUDE IS KEY

Gratitude is the key that unlocks and opens doors to healing. Gratitude gives you the power and ability to change your perception, quicken inspiration, and move you toward action that will benefit and aid you in an instant.

In July of 2002, I was sitting in the doctor's office with my husband, waiting for the test results from an MRI. The doctor came in and read the last part of the report to us. The results were conclusive for Multiple Sclerosis. When I received that diagnosis, my thoughts were not the typical "Oh no!" or "Why me?" or "My life is over" sort of thoughts. Instead, and almost audibly, I remember the very first thought that came into my mind was "I am just grateful I'm not going crazy! There is actually a reason I feel this crummy." I didn't know it then, but having that one simple thought of gratitude, be the first thought that went through my mind set me on the path of healing from that moment forward.

Gratitude is a perception changer. If I were to take 5 people and stand them side by side, then play out a scenario right in front of them, immediately separate them into different rooms, and ask them to tell me what they just witnessed, I would get 5 different stories. Perception is tricky this way. There is no right or wrong, good or bad, just differences. Differences in backgrounds, life experiences, what each had for lunch, or how much sleep they got the night before. There are so many things that play into our individual viewpoints. The beauty in this is that there are also many different options. Yay for options! If I don't like what I see, then maybe all it takes is to choose another way to look at it.

Have you ever felt desperate, helpless, hopeless, or stuck in your life, with seemingly no way to change things, no way out? I have. Many times. Maybe you are what I call an "obstacle thinker." An obstacle thinker is someone who is great at finding all the reasons why something can't be done, focusing on every obstacle that seems to be in their way. Gratitude is the quickest way I know to pull yourself out of these types of feelings, to shift your perspective, thereby changing your thoughts about a situation. Inspiration can come into your mind and through your heart in the form of thoughts or feelings. When you are thinking or feeling from a place of desperation, helplessness, hopelessness, or feeling stuck, it's like trying to pour inspiration through the small side of an upside down funnel. It is difficult, discouraging, and mostly unsuccessful. You turn the funnel around using gratitude. Then the funnel is open and the inspiration flows into your mind and heart effortlessly. Being in the flow of inspiration is truly magical and transforming.

Now that inspiring ideas, feelings of hope, and options are flowing to you, your next step is to act upon that inspiration. Leave no room for doubt or second guessing, or talking yourself out of it. Just do it! The action you feel inspired to do may seem completely irrelevant to aiding you or your circumstances. As long as it is legal and moral, you can't mess it up. Trust me, just do it a couple of times and see what happens. This is the adventure part of your journey. It is learning to believe in yourself and your ability to change your current circumstances. It moves you into creating something new and different. It is FUN!

This is an exercise I have people do in my classes. It takes approximately 15 minutes.

1-Get a piece of paper and something to write with.

2-Write down the 3 greatest challenges you are experiencing in your life.

3-Choose the one that is driving you nuts, that gnaws at you, and write it down again.

4-Now write down 3 things that you can be grateful for about that challenge. Give yourself a 10 minute time limit so your brain doesn't take an escape route.

Remember that the whole direction of a potentially crippling disease was altered by the single thought: "I am just grateful I'm not going crazy!" I have had people look at me like I am crazy when I ask them to do this exercise. Yes, you can find 3 things to be grateful for. A little trick to do if you are struggling to write anything down, is to place your pen on the paper and don't lift the pen off until you begin writing something.

_____

_____

_____

_____

_____

_____

_____

_____

_____

_____

_____

_____

_____

_____

What just happened for you? Did your perspective shift? Do you feel a little lighter, maybe more hopeful about the challenge you are facing? Are there ideas coming to your mind? Are there action steps you can take? This, and so much more, is possible just by simply applying gratitude to your challenges.

I love this exercise because as I teach this principle in classes, a shift takes place in the energy of the room that is palpable to everyone. It is always amazing to see people's faces light up and their bodies begin to relax as stress is released. They feel empowered to do something about their life, and circumstances, even if only in small measure at first. I love it, I love it, I love it!

I have taken this gratitude exercise and shortened it to apply it to everyday circumstances. I don't always have the time or pen and paper to write things down, so I will just think about at least one thing to be grateful for in that given moment. If someone or something presents itself as a problem, I first acknowledge in my mind that the place they are coming from is different than the place I am coming from. Then I apply gratitude about them or the situation quickly. It is that simple.

FORGIVENESS IS POWERFUL

I love the power that comes to me when I practice forgiveness daily; especially forgiving myself for the things I inaccurately think or feel about myself. I have come to understand how damaging it is to the health of my body, mind, and spirit to carry around unnecessary burdens. I can give my burdens over to a higher power; and by doing so, I heal and gain an increased capacity to love myself and others.

Forgiveness of others and myself is an important step in the process of healing for me. Sometimes forgiving someone I feel has wronged me or harmed me in some way is easier for me than forgiving myself.

I developed false belief patterns as I moved through life. For example: the belief that I would be more righteous if I held on to mistakes, or that beating myself up mentally over a perceived wrong I committed would somehow make it better. Instead it made me sick. Another example of those beliefs was that I felt I needed to suffer somehow and that would make it all right. It never did. It only made things worse and drove me further into depression and illness. There was the guilt and shame aspect to it as well.

Guilt is an emotion that is destructive on many levels. Guilt and shame are damaging to the mind, body, and spirit when you allow those emotions to hang around for any length of time. Guilt is only useful for one thing and that is to let you know that something is out of balance in your life and it needs to be looked at and adjusted- that is it. I had forgiveness all backwards for a long time. I over complicated and underestimated the power of its ability to heal until…

I have had two near death experiences. The following took place during the first experience. I found myself having a conversation with Jesus Christ. Conversing was done through thoughts and was very easy and devoid of awkwardness in any way. I found Him to be very, very loving, warm and compassionate. He spoke with me as a best friend would, as a brother would. We were just chatting for a minute and then He asked me two very poignant questions- questions that caused me to pause then and sometimes even now. He asked me "Why do you beat yourself up?" and "Why is the Atonement not good enough for you?"

I remember a pause, my pause, and a complete lack of thought or feeling on my part. I became answerless. In my mind I was thinking, "I don't know" and in that moment of Jesus asking me great questions, I had an "aha" moment, and we both laughed a little at my own silliness.

He proceeded to teach me about forgiveness, about the ability to let things go and to let God fill in the holes that I could not. He taught me how carrying around burdens and past errors was unnecessary and how forgiving would ease my burden and lighten my load. He taught me about the "sin" of not letting it go and not forgiving, especially forgiving myself because that is where I struggled most. The word "sin" in this case is meant to explain the harm that comes to our mind, body, and soul when we hang on to guilt or shame. I don't know about you, but sometimes I swear I wear guilt and shame like a badge of honor. It is ridiculous! As far as forgiving others, Christ taught me that forgiving other people is really a selfish act, and this is not a negative thing. Forgiveness isn't about the other person. It is about you.

How many rocks do you carry around from day to day? Let's use this illustration: Take an empty backpack and put it on your back. You are going to wear it throughout the day. As your day progresses, things happen. Your boss accuses you of doing something you didn't do and you get reprimanded. You have an argument with your spouse and the issue doesn't get resolved. Someone is unkind to your child and gets away with it. There are hurt feelings between you and your parents or your in-laws. Someone borrows something from you and doesn't return it. Someone hurts you unintentionally, or intentionally. You get called names or ugly gossip is spread about you. These are small examples that can occur day to day. What if something really tragic occurs as a result of someone's neglect, bad behavior, or ill will toward another? Events such as abuse, death, crime against others etc. would perhaps require even larger stones be put in the pack, however the process of healing is the same.

Now add in a few rocks for the self-punishment and loathing you do each day- "I'm stupid, fat, unworthy, not good enough, lazy, or unacceptable." In a very short period of time the weight can become overwhelming, burdensome, and heavy. Have you ever heard you or someone else say, "I feel overwhelmed", "I'm so depressed", or "I feel like the weight of the world is on my shoulders"? It is more likely than not that there are a lot of rocks piled up in that backpack and there needs to be some serious emptying going on.

If I choose to hang on to anger, resentment, bitterness and envy, the only person I am harming is me. The person who committed the offense against me isn't being punished by their mistake when I hang on to it, I am. How crazy is that logic?

Jesus wanted me to let it go, He wants me to let it go. If I choose to hang on to all of those rocks it will clutter up my mind with debris, weigh heavily on my body, and crush my soul. Why, oh why, would I choose that? He taught me that the forgiveness process is really quite simple and that there is no need to make it a long drawn out process. He said He is able to make things right, to put things into balance, where I am unable to. Jesus is a powerful, loving, healing being who desires for each of us to experience the healing aspect of forgiveness in our lives.

By practicing forgiveness and turning it over to a higher power, you can actually feel the load lighten, and see the burden lifted in your eyes and on the faces of others. Forgiveness is very life affirming and does wonders for your health and well-being. I have seen it happen over and over with family and with clients I work with.

A few years ago I heard about a man whose practice was centered on stress management, with forgiveness being a key piece. My oldest son became ill with ulcerative colitis and inside I knew it was not just a physical issue. I knew there were emotional issues tied in with it as well. I called the office of this man and scheduled an appointment. His office was a 4 hour drive from where we lived. We drove down and spent 2 hours with him then we drove back home. The time I spent with him was eye opening. He also taught about the simplicity of forgiveness, even in a "fake it till you make it sort of way," if you had to.

Forgiveness isn't fake, but sometimes when you feel particularly hurt by someone's words or actions against you, the fake it part comes in very handy until it becomes genuine. I was given a simple daily exercise that I could use. My brain thought that forgiveness had to be complicated, (yes, even after my near death experience) so of course I was a bit skeptical, but I had driven all that way and paid a significant amount of money to hear this advice, so I decided I'd better give it a try.

This is the activity I was given and he suggested that I do it daily. I should say out loud, "I forgive (insert name) for (insert grievance)," then, "I forgive myself for (insert any negative emotion you are feeling toward that person, situation or yourself)." You then ask God to forgive them or yourself. Please keep in mind that you are to do this when you are alone without people within earshot, and especially never to the face of the person you are forgiving. That would lead to all kinds of other problems. It was suggested I could even do it while I was showering; 1-I do it daily, 2-I'm by myself, and 3- I could let all the negative emotions and feelings just wash off of me and go down the drain. Picture the person in front of you when you do this. See them nodding and accepting your forgiveness. This activity may seem trivial or too simple to do any good at all, but it really does work.

These simple concepts may fly in the face of certain religious beliefs. Please remember that these are my experiences. I share them only in the hope that someone else may be able to apply them and gain peace and healing for themselves and their relationships by my doing so. The Mayo Clinic reports the health benefits from forgiving can include:

- Healthier relationships
- Greater spiritual and psychological well-being
- Less anxiety and stress
- Lower blood pressure
- Fewer symptoms of depression
- Stronger immune system
- Improved heart health
- Higher self esteem

I've heard it said: "Forgiveness is a gift you give yourself." And I agree completely.

EATING AND MOVING

"You are what you eat." I used to not take that saying seriously. I do now! I used to make excuses for making poor eating choices, such as "It doesn't really matter or just a 'little' sugar, soda or fried food isn't a big deal." Turns out it is a big deal. When you are trying to get out of pain and heal a chronic illness, or take preventative measures to avoid disease in the first place, it matters! Eating unprocessed, non-GMO, organic food is important.

From the time I was a little girl I was taught in small, everyday ways about food, herbs, and supplements. I remember being at my great-grandparents home, in their large garden out back. My cousin Linda and

I would go out and pick carrots, raspberries, peas, and tomatoes from the garden, then take them into the house to be washed and eaten. My great-grandfather, Leland Barnes, came over and showed me and my husband the best way to plant tomato starters one year, early on in our marriage.

My father's parents had a beautiful garden that always included a lot of chard. My mother's parents had a small orchard with apricot, cherry, apple, pear, and plum trees. My mother and grandmothers always grew herbs in their gardens.

When I was young, my cousin and I would sleep over at my grandparents and sometimes she would give us clear capsules and a bowl full of goldenseal herb powder and we would sit and fill the capsules. I had no idea at the time what goldenseal was, it was just fun to fill the capsules. I would catch snippets of conversations about this home remedy or that new/old supplement. My grandfather and father hunted deer and elk, and we spent a lot of time fishing for trout every summer. I am the oldest of seven children, and we rarely ate out when I was growing up. We had dinner together nearly every night. Both of my parents cooked and so did I. My mother taught me how to bottle fruits, vegetables, and juices, and we canned every late summer through early fall. Yes, I had it pretty good growing up. I have always loved fruits and vegetables, probably because I had access to them as a child.

Using food and herbs for medicinal and nutritional purposes is second nature to me. I simply wandered away from that as my life changed and got more hectic in my early married and young mom years. Fast food and convenience food crept in, and bottling my own fruits and vegetables faded away. I didn't completely abandon everything I knew, but it did get put on the back burner in a lot of ways.

Going back to my story in the beginning of this book, I knew that when I gave up all of those medications, I was going to need to wake up that part of my brain that had been lulled into laziness about nutrition. That part of me needed to become conscious again. I knew there had to be answers. What could I do to support my body, to effect change and begin the healing process, utilizing nutrition? Let me be clear about this. It wasn't as if I just received a huge 'aha' about everything I needed to eat or what supplements to use. It came to me piece by piece and step by step. It is a journey I am still on today, 12 years later. It is one of the reasons I became a health coach. I have studied, read, listened to lectures, and attended classes about nutrition to the extent that my husband believes there can't possibly be anything else on this subject for me to learn. I'm joking (a little) about that. There is always more to learn.

The color green is my favorite nutritional color. Green is the color of healing, and the color of life in nature. Green foods are highly alkalizing for the body. And no, green food coloring doesn't count. I have always enjoyed leafy greens. My grandparents and parents grew chard and beets with their yummy, leafy green tops in their gardens so, of course, I love them. Now I enjoy green smoothies. I use dehydrated greens for smoothies because I cannot always get enough using spinach, kale, and other greens by themselves, and I also occasionally juice greens as well. One of my favorite juices to do is:
- 1 pineapple
- 1 bunch of parsley
- 1 apple
- ¼ inch piece of ginger.

I also like to put a bit of parsley with a pineapple spear and juice them together; it just seems to make the juice better.

Wheatgrass is another power packed super food. I also use a chlorophyll supplement in my water, especially if the water is unfiltered. There is a list of products I use in the back of this book.

I made the decision three years ago to be vegetarian. I have had periods of time where I have been vegan and also had raw, living foods only. All have been beneficial and I don't ascribe to any one way of eating all the time, except I do not eat meat any more. Meat is highly acidic to the body, and disease and illness thrive in an acidic environment. The hormones and diets fed to most of the animals we consume these days are harmful in many ways to our bodies as well.

Creating a balance between acidity and alkalinity is very important for our overall health and wellbeing. It is more difficult for disease to thrive in an alkaline environment. This is one of the reasons why greens are such an important part of my diet. Drinking good water is also an important part of this equation. I avoid sodas, sugars, artificial sweeteners, and high fructose corn syrups. Water, water, and more water. Learn to love it! If you're hooked on other drinks, take steps to wean yourself off by substituting water at least once a day for the other options. This won't take long to do and your taste buds will adjust. I enjoy squeezing a lemon or lime into my water. You can also add cucumber slices, berries, ginger and mint to flavor water. If you are a heavy coffee drinker, consider alternating with good quality teas. Tea can be less acidic than coffee. On the next page is a chart showing you the different pH levels of foods when they are eaten.

I try to purchase organic vegetables and fruits. I used to think I couldn't afford to buy organic. I now say I can't afford not to. Toxic pesticides used on our food supply are harmful for our bodies and those toxins can build up over time. Here is a simple inexpensive fruit/vegetable wash to use on produce before you eat it.

Fill a sink with Clean Water; add White Vinegar, (3 parts water, 1 part vinegar) and stir. Add fruits and vegetables and soak for 10 minutes. The water will be dirty and the wax and chemicals on the produce will be removed. It is best to use purified water, and for the produce to be at room temperature. Then rinse and let the produce air dry when finished.

pH = Potential for Health

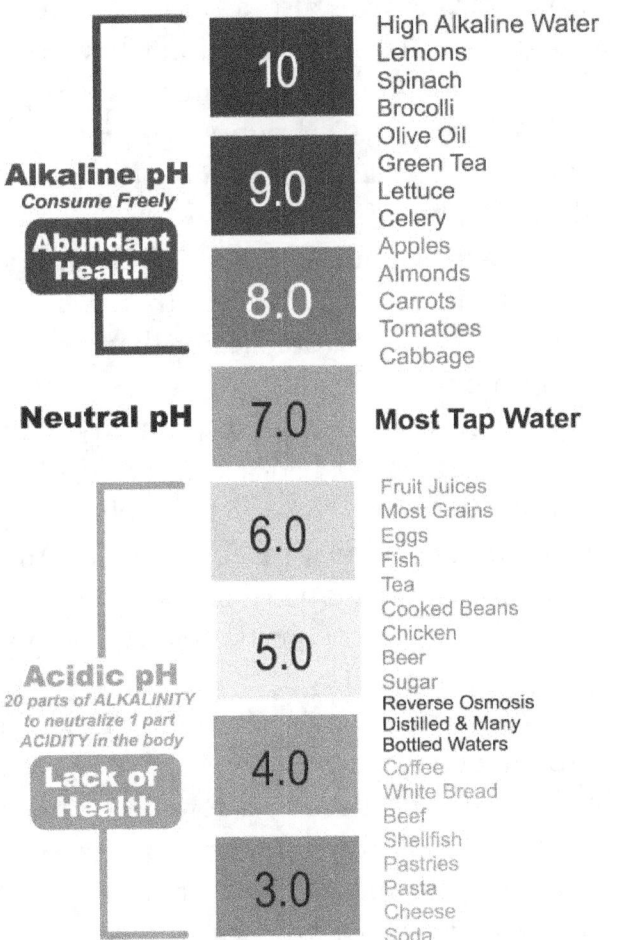

Alkaline pH *Consume Freely* **Abundant Health**	10	High Alkaline Water Lemons Spinach Brocolli Olive Oil Green Tea
	9.0	Lettuce Celery Apples
	8.0	Almonds Carrots Tomatoes Cabbage
Neutral pH	7.0	**Most Tap Water**
	6.0	Fruit Juices Most Grains Eggs Fish Tea
Acidic pH *20 parts of ALKALINITY to neutralize 1 part ACIDITY in the body* **Lack of Health**	5.0	Cooked Beans Chicken Beer Sugar **Reverse Osmosis Distilled & Many Bottled Waters**
	4.0	Coffee White Bread Beef Shellfish
	3.0	Pastries Pasta Cheese Soda

Our health depends on the food, drink and lifestyle choices we make on a daily basis.

I am a big fan of farmers markets. Our bodies thrive on a diet that is indigenous to our environment. If it is locally grown chances are your body will thank you for it. Local farmers are also a great resource for those of you who either don't have or are lacking in the green thumb department. When you eat bright, vibrant, fresh vegetables and fruits, your body will be more bright, vibrant, and healthy.

When it comes to food and nutrition, what you put inside your body has a much greater effect on your health than anything you do on the outside.

When was the last time you sat down in a quiet place and had a conversation with your body? Have you ever? Maybe you are laughing at the idea of doing such a thing. Actually, it can be very amusing and even funny to listen to your body talk, and given the chance, it will!

Get a pen and notebook or journal. Go sit outside somewhere, or find a quiet place indoors. Take in a few deep breaths. Breathe in through your nose and out through your mouth. Now set the intention in your mind that you will receive specific answers from your body regarding whatever health challenge you may be dealing with. It may be about your weight, an illness, pain, a lack of energy, anything. Next ask your body the question, "What can I do to support you?" Listen and write down whatever comes to you. Trust it. It may be a single thought or an entire conversation that occurs. Just have fun with it!

_____

_____

_____

_____

_____

_____

_____

_____

_____

_____

_____

_____

_____

As a former fitness trainer, I have tried almost every form of exercise there is. One of the reasons I think I have been able to avoid succumbing to muscle deterioration or a decline in coordination that often occurs with MS is because of the variety of physical activities I engage in. Ultimately, the most important aspect of physical activity is to just do it! Choose a couple of activities you enjoy and do them regularly. Walking is a great place to begin; it's inexpensive, available, and super beneficial. I enjoy strength training for my muscles, biking for aerobics, an exercise ball works for balance, and mini trampoline to get my lymph nodes going. Yoga is a great way to improve flexibility, connect with your inner self, and learn breathing techniques. Once again, have fun! If you aren't, then you're not going to stick with it. If you have a social personality, get a workout buddy, take classes, or participate in outdoor activities or team sports.

Our bodies are magnificent, intelligent, and miraculous. The body knows how to heal itself. When you get a cut, the body knows it needs to cleanse the wound by bleeding, and then slow down the bleeding by thickening the blood and scabbing over the wound. I know that's the kindergarten version, but you understand what I mean. I don't sit there and tell my body step by step what to do, it just knows.

Nutrition and physical activity are both important pieces in my being able to live a life without symptoms of chronic illness. That doesn't mean that I don't succumb to the occasional cold or flu, although when I do, it is short lived. What it does mean is that I get to live. I get to live free of symptoms. I get to live without medications and the nasty side effects from them. I get to live a healthy, happy, and fulfilling life. All because I choose to drink a little more water, exercise, and support my body by eating a diet rich in nutritious vegetables and fruits. These are simple things I can do that lead to great results for the health and wellness of my body.

PINECONES AND PLAYTIME

How long has it been since you played like a kid? When was the last time you played a game, or participated in an activity you enjoyed as a child? Are you all grown up, forgetting about the child inside of you longing to come out and play?

Children look for, and see the possibilities in everything. Their imaginations run wild. They have a "can do" attitude. You fasten a towel around their shoulders like a cape and suddenly they can fly! You place a large spoon in a child's hand and they turn into a rock star singing and dancing like they're on stage. Give a child paints or a box of crayons and they'll create a masterpiece. They have wonder and hope and believe in life and all of its possibilities. How often do we visit that place in our hearts and minds as adults? I am not suggesting you live in Fantasyland; however I have found childlike play to be a vital principle to my healing. I suggest you do something you enjoy daily, even if for just a few minutes.

Childlike energy is infectious. It's fun and contagious. This is something you want to catch! When you are feeling uninspired, sad, down, stuck, or frazzled, do something a child would do. Play pat-a-cake, dance, or go outside and twirl in circles. Watch your attitude and energy shift, quickly. If you are so grown up you can't figure out how, or you are too embarrassed to be childlike, then watch an infant or child, play peek-a-boo, or copy what they do. If they are blowing spit bubbles, then you do it too. Granted this does not help with the embarrassment part, but get over yourself! Have you ever seen adults interacting with babies? We all look stupid, but who cares? The rewards are solid. Have you ever wondered how a small baby can captivate and hold the attention of an adult, even a group of adults? What do you feel when you are looking at or holding a child when they are asleep? Words like peaceful, sweet, carefree, comforting, and love come to my mind. This is why it is so important to do things that remind us of a simpler, more carefree time in our life. It is inspiring and freeing to let your inner child come out and play. Play with your children, or with other adults, or even be your own best friend! You are important, the child within you is important.

When I was a child, my family had a tradition of going to Yellowstone National Park every summer. My family included great-grandparents, grandparents, my aunt and uncle, cousins, my parents, and siblings. The adults did a lot of fishing, cooking, setting up trailers and camp. We kids found ways to entertain ourselves. My cousin Linda and I would wander around the campground collecting pinecones of all varieties. We would gather up a whole bunch and then we would create playhouses with them by laying them out in blueprint fashion making "rooms" to play in. We had wild imaginations and would create all sorts of stories about who we were, and the lives we were pretending to live inside those pinecone walls. Two of our younger sisters opted to use the outhouses as their playhouses. I still can't figure that one out, but oh well! Now the adult in me might be tempted to think things like "I'm too tired. Picking up all those pinecones will take forever. That is a silly idea."

Getting into your play energy, your creative, fun, carefree energy is healing to your body and soul. Suggestions for activities to bring out your inner child:

- Ride a bicycle
- Hopscotch
- Blow bubbles
- Collect rocks
- Read a favorite book from your youth
- Build a snowman/snow fort
- Ice skating
- Play-Doh or clay
- Jump rope
- Play cards "Go Fish" or "Crazy 8's"
- Swing
- Slide
- Play in a sandbox
- Sidewalk chalk
- Dance
- Lie on a blanket outside and find pictures in the clouds
- Blow dandelions and make a wish
- Play in the soap suds when you wash dishes
- Frisbee

- Hula Hoop
- Build with blocks/Tinker toys
- Play dress up
- Have a tea party
- Color in a coloring book with crayons
- Play tag, kick the can, statue, or no bears are out tonight with the neighbors
- Climb a tree
- Fingerpaint
- Skip instead of walk
- Play jacks

These are just a few of the things that I did as a child. Now, as an adult, I do things for myself too. I call it self-care. This is similar to embracing my inner child, yet different. There is purpose and good in doing both. Self-care consists of things such as:

- Getting a massage
- Meditation
- Detox bath
- Calling a friend
- Listening to music
- Taking a drive up the canyon
- Playing a game
- Watching a good movie
- Sitting in an infrared sauna

- A nap
- Laughing/crying
- Get a foot-zone treatment
- Riding my bicycle

It is important to take care of yourself. It is important to embrace the childlike wonder within you and also to take care of the adult you are now. Love yourself, take care of yourself, and create health in your life. You matter!

CHANGING YOUR STORY

What is your story? What are the stories of your ancestors? Your parents? Your grandparents? Are the stories filled with struggle, suffering, or sacrifice? I know mine are. When I look back at my heritage, I see immense struggle, suffering, and sacrifice. There were great challenges with money, war, and health, the same stories also include bits about greatness, how righteous or noble they were, and how revered they were. Were they heroes because of the intensity or duration of their struggles and sacrifices? This is where our perspectives can get twisted or mixed up. I have come to understand that my subconscious may take on the belief that struggle + sacrifice + suffering = heroism, nobility, and righteousness. So in a mixed up way we begin to create scenarios in our own life that make us heroes who are noble and righteous, through our self-made struggle and sacrifice.

We want to be the hero. We want to gain rewards in heaven, and there is a desire to be appreciated for our service and sacrifices. About now you may be thinking this is ridiculous nonsense! And you would be correct. To our conscious mind it is silly. However, the belief in our subconscious mind is saying, "Yep! That makes sense."

So we create an identity around being ill. We identify ourselves with the disease. We identify ourselves with the struggle. When our identity gets wrapped up in the illness, it becomes a roadblock in our journey to healing. Who are you with the disease? Who are you without it? Are you enough? Are you good enough without it? It seems as though we spend a lot of our time and energy thinking or feeling that we aren't 'good enough'. Consequently, we can get caught up in having to prop ourselves up by seeking attention, gaining our self-worth from outside sources, rather than within. We attempt to get this validation through sacrifice, suffering and struggle.

People give you attention, sympathy, and prop you up by telling you how good you are and how strong you are for enduring all that you are going through. If even a part of you is feeling some self-worth in it, it can cause a reluctance to heal, for who are you without it? Who will validate you if it is healed? This is where you get to become the hero in your own story. You get to change your beliefs about who you are and who you are not with chronic illness. Change your story. Change your life.

My story goes a little something like this: My body is a gift. I am responsible for my health and happiness, no one else. My body functions beautifully. My body communicates with me, and lets me know when it needs support. It may signal me through illness, pain, or fatigue, that something is out of alignment. The symptoms of disease I once had have been replaced with vitality. Drug therapies have been replaced with natural therapies and nutrition. I feel joy and peace, even amidst my challenges. I love my body and I am grateful for all that it does for me every day. I love my healthy, happy, amazing life! I am the hero in my own story.

One last way I would like to offer as a tool for healing your life, and even your heritage, is through energy healing. Energy healing aids not only us, but can also help us clear up problems that were passed down to us from our ancestors. I found energy work in 2007. It was new to me, yet something in my soul nudged me to find out more. My introduction to energy healing was the Simply Healed method, founded by Carolyn Cooper. I have said many times that I am grateful this was the first modality I was exposed to. It is just as the name suggests, simple and healing. I learned how to not only create healing for myself and my children, but also how to heal things for my ancestors through me. This may sound weird, or strange, but it is actually very cool, and I have had several special experiences helping my loved ones who have passed on clear up their issues. Simply Healed helps clear the negative emotions on all levels. It was very instrumental for me near the beginning of my journey to healing, and it continues to bless my life today. I have since become certified in the Quantum Touch and Reiki modalities. I have a love for these methods as well. There are many loving, powerful healers and many modalities of Energy Healing available. I encourage you to find practitioners where you live and try it out. It has made a huge difference in my life, for the better.

I've received many gifts from this experience in my life. It helped me see how my life, as it was, wasn't working for me. I recognized the amount of stress I had buried myself under, and was able to change it. It taught me to find answers within, to listen to and trust my intuition, not discount and dismiss it. My compassion for people with chronic illness has grown.

It helped me learn to enjoy the simple things in life: the beauty of a sunset, nature and its wonders, the sound of laughter, especially my own, and the ability to laugh at myself and not take myself too seriously.

I know that I have options. If I don't like the circumstances I find myself in, then I at the very least can choose how to perceive it. I have learned to be grateful in ways I never considered before. I have a greater appreciation for health, even for my challenges with it. I learned how nutrition and food can help me or hurt me, and now make conscious, informed decisions about what I eat.

I learned God is good, that people are good, that I am good. It's taught me how we all do the best we know how, and that our hearts are generally good and loving. We are not left alone on this earth. It only takes one spark to light up a dark space.

I have learned there is more than one way to fix a problem, and nature has many things to assist us, such as essential oils, herbs, food, plants, trees, and animals. And perhaps, most importantly, I have learned to find the value and gifts in all of the experiences in my life.

Now you get to write your story. What do you want to create with your health? What do you want to change about your life? Write your story. Write as if it's already happening. Then tell your new story.

Your New Story

_____

_____

_____

_____

_____

_____

_____

_____

_____

_____

_____

_____

_____

_____

_____

_____

_____

ABOUT THE AUTHOR

Your health opens the door for you to live the life you want. My goal is assisting you in igniting your own magic and healing abilities. When you're struggling and suffering through life, accepting that's just the way it is, it leaves you in bondage to the disease.

Challenge your beliefs about what is possible with this experience for you. I DID! I took charge of my life and my health- **all** components of my health, mental, emotional, spiritual, and physical.

I live a freer, happier, healthier life than any doctor told me was possible. What is possible for you? I am here to support your journey to healing and health, and have created a community to support you too, because you do not have to do this alone.

I invite you to take your next step to take back your health and your life. Go to LoriTidwell.com

www.ingramcontent.com/pod-product-compliance
Lightning Source LLC
Chambersburg PA
CBHW062109280526
45788CB00003B/1405